I0435389

Fybromyalgia Relief Guide

Signs and Symptoms of Fibromyalgia and

Natural Treatments for Fibromyalgia

Table of Contents

Introduction

This book contains important information on Fibromyalgia and the signs and symptoms related to the condition. It also provides you with useful strategies that have been used by many to help deal with Fibromyalgia without resorting to medication. These are methods that even therapists employ as the main means of treating Fibromyalgia and are sometimes suggested to be used alongside other treatments.

Hopefully, by the end of this book, you will have enough information to help you or your loved ones cope with and eventually overcome Fibromyalgia the natural way.

Chapter 1 – Fibromyalgia: What Is It?

Fibromyalgia is a problem suffered by many without them even knowing they have it. The problem lies with the confusing nature of the condition. Add to this the surprising number of people who deny it exists – a good lot of them coming from the medical field itself. However, for those who have Fibromyalgia, the grief and pain it causes is all too real, so it is necessary to deal with the condition right away. In solving any problem, one must start by asking the all-important first questions.

What is Fibromyalgia?

The term Fibromyalgia (FM) is derived from three words – *"fibro"* (Latin), *"myo"* and *"algia"* (both Greek). Roughly translated together, it actually means connective tissue and muscle pain. This gives you a rough description of what sufferers of Fibromyalgia experience. Persons in the medical field give a more detailed summary. They characterize it as muscle pain and/or pressure sensitivity of the muscles. Such pain and sensitivity is widespread. It is also chronic or recurring.

Though pain is the most prominent symptom of Fibromyalgia, it is not the only one. In fact, there are several symptoms and such symptoms may vary from one patient to another. As a result, some experts refer to the condition as Fibromyalgia Syndrome (FMS). The significance of calling it a syndrome points to the fact that it is actually a conglomeration of numerous signs and symptoms caused by a single condition. This affects diagnosis as it recognizes that not all cases of FMS are alike. There will be varying symptoms and varying degrees of intensity of such.

While the debate as to what to call Fibromyalgia does not affect patients much, there is still a surprising few who question the existence of the condition altogether. You have to remember that Fibromyalgia is a real medical condition and if you have been diagnosed with it, you can attest to the realness of the pain it causes. Do not be dissuaded by doctors and persons who say it is all in your head.

The fact is that Fibromyalgia Syndrome has been confirmed and classified by several experts around the world. In America, it is classified as a disorder which affects a person's nervous system. Based on present research, the symptoms of the condition are caused by a malfunction of the central nervous system in processing pain signals. In essence, the person is experiencing inexplicable pain and sensitivity because the nervous system is telling the rest of the body that it is in pain though it really is not.

What are the Signs and Symptoms?

To be able to cope with Fibromyalgia, it is best for you to be aware of the major manifestations of this medical condition. The following are the major symptoms:

- **Pain**

This symptom is in the name of the condition itself. As such, it is the main symptom of FMS. This pain is not just any ordinary pain, however. The criteria for FMS related pain is threefold. These are:

1. Widespread and Migrating Pain

    You will often hear people with Fibromyalgia say that they feel pain everywhere, and they are not exaggerating. The nature of FMS related pain is that it is widespread and in many cases, it even moves from one place to another. The pain may also be accompanied by muscle spasms or stiffness. It affects both the muscles and the joints or connective tissues in between.

    Patients often describe it as the feeling of being beat up, as if they were hit hard in several places, causing pain and soreness of their muscles to the touch. It is as if they have several bruises all over. Others compare it to the pain of having lifted heavy weight. Their muscles feel so overworked to the point of pain and sensitivity. It is also noted to be a radiating pain and can easily be confused as arthritis or just plain fatigue.

2. Inexplicable Pain

    The pain related to Fibromyalgia is that which cannot be attributed to any apparent source. There are no bruises, scratches and strain. Doctors may attempt to find an explanation for the pain such as bone breakage, internal bruising, or any one of the usual suspects. However, they usually find nothing. You may think the pain is all in your head, and you might not be entirely wrong.

The pain is actually due to a signal mix-up in your nervous system. Your brain and nerves are telling you that you feel pain, though there is no logical source of it. Somewhere between your nerves and your brain, confusion ensues as to what signals are being fired. Unfortunately, your brain interprets the said signals as pain.

3. Recurring or Chronic Pain

The problem most people with FMS have is that the pain they feel always seems to be there. There are times when it seems to go away, but it always comes back. Another attribute of this pain is that it seems to vary in intensity from excruciating to tolerable. It is basically impossible to predict.

- **"Fibro-Fog"**

Another prominent symptom of Fibromyalgia is the confusion that comes with it. It has been nicknamed "Mental Fog" or "Fibro-Fog". This basically describes what happens to the mental faculties of a person with FMS. Their mind goes foggy, their memory becomes unreliable, they cannot concentrate well and they become inexplicably confused. In worst cases, sufferers become flustered by everyday tasks such as arranging their work desks or even preparing their food. It leads to frustration, stress and even depression. This adds another level of pain, one that is mental and emotional. The confusion also comes and goes just like the fatigue and pain. This symptom is attributed to the same malfunction of the central nervous system. The misfiring signals create a seeming cognitive distortion. It is like an overt manifestation of the confusion happening on the cellular level within your body.

- **Fatigue**

  Aside from the pain, those with FMS also seem to suffer from bouts of inexplicable fatigue. They often feel as if they had just run a marathon or had just lifted hundreds of pounds. The level of fatigue they feel is so extreme, but is also seemingly without reason. More often than not, those who have FMS do not feel well enough to do any heavy lifting or strenuous activity anyway. So the fatigue they feel is just as bizarre as the pain they have. This can easily be confused with the symptoms of another disorder called Chronic Fatigue Syndrome. However, if the other mentioned symptoms are present, FMS is the more likely culprit.

- **Being Sensitive to Weather**

  Many of those who have FMS have said that they feel that they are weather sensitive. That is, they know when a chill is coming or an increase of temperature is imminent. They even say they can predict it before the weather man on television says so. This may seem far-fetched to most, but experts suggest that this is actually a real manifestation of the condition. Our body truly is sensitive to slight changes in temperature, but most of us do not notice this because our bodies normally react more to sudden or drastic changes. For those with FMS however, their nervous systems are not functioning as they should. As a result, minor changes in temperature or weather which your body would normally let you ignore can get confused for pain signals.

Most who claim to be weather sensitive have indeed related the same to pain. They claim to know when a storm is coming because they literally feel it in the form of a growing pain or even feeling of fatigue. Others may also include depression as a manifestation of this sensitivity. However, this is more likely attributable to another condition altogether. Some who have been treated for FMS have reported that relocation to places where the weather is milder has improved their condition, but it does not seem to work for everyone.

- **Trouble Getting Some Sleep**

  Most, if not all, of those who suffer from FMS have trouble sleeping. The inability to sleep is most likely caused by the pain associated with Fibromyalgia, but it is also possible that it is associated with your malfunctioning central nervous system. Whichever is the case, lack of sleep is never good for anyone. It is even worse for those with Fibromyalgia. A constant sleep deficit can easily amplify all the aforementioned symptoms as well as cause other medical conditions altogether. It can worsen the "fibro-fog" and make you less prepared to deal with the pain and fatigue brought upon by your condition. Sleeping disorders can be treated separately from FMS to help you cope better and you should ask your doctor about your options.

Chapter 2 – Going Natural

Why Go Natural?

While many who sell alternative and "natural" remedies might tell you that you should go natural because it is safer, there is no actual evidence to support this. In fact, some of the remedies considered natural such as herbs can also be dangerous when taken alongside other medication or substances. Some chemical components of natural remedies are also dangerous in improper quantities. The reality is that you will likely have to consult your doctor about natural remedies much like other medication if you want to be absolutely sure that what you are taking or using is safe.

So this then begs the question, why would you want to go natural in the first place?

The answer is actually simple – certain natural remedies just work. This does not mean that natural remedies are the miracle cure for FMS and other conditions; it simply means that some natural remedies such as herbs and oils have been used with a degree of success by some physicians, therapists and do-it-yourself patients. The fact remains that medical science has not yet completely understood FMS and this opens the door for several alternative forms of treatment that can eventually become part of mainstream medicine, as our understanding of the condition widens and medical science advances.

A Word of Warning

Remember, the fact that the remedies in the following sections (and chapters) are "natural" does not mean they do not come with their dangers. If used improperly, they can pose risks to your health. Take the time to ask your doctor about them. Do not simply rely on the salesperson's pitch or the store clerk's advice. Do not be afraid or embarrassed to suggest these treatments to your physician. The fact is several doctors and therapists actually encourage the use of these alternative forms of treatment alongside or as a part of FMS treatment. Ask them if the alternative treatment is compatible with any other treatment or medication you are on to avoid any untoward incidents. Though these remedies have already been tested by some doctors and patients, their effects may vary based on you predisposition.

With that being said, here are some natural remedies for your consideration:

Using Herbs

These herbs are particularly used by therapists to help persons with FMS cope with the insomnia that comes along with the condition. They can also help dull the pain and fatigue felt due to FMS. Take note of their uses and pay close attention to the side effects indicated.

- **Melatonin**

  This is a supplement derived from herbs that is similar to the melatonin being produced by your own body. Your pineal gland found in your brain produces this substance and is used for regulation of your sleeping cycles. It is a remedy often used to fight jetlag.

Possible side effects: Headaches

- **Valerian**

This is an herb that has been in use since the time of ancient Greece. It is used as a sedative and is one of the predecessors of modern sedatives. Generally, it is only safe to use for up to four weeks. Some go up to six weeks, but it is best to consult a doctor first.

Possible side effects: Headaches, dizziness and upset stomach

- **Chamomile**

This is a common herb which is taken as a tea. It is well known for its sedative effects and is often suggested by some doctors for that exact purpose.

Possible side effects: Decreases clotting of blood (not advised for those taking blood thinners)

- **Echinacea**

This is an herb which is very popular for those with FMS. It is not used to treat pain or insomnia; instead it is known for its use in relieving fatigue. A study conducted on FMS patients using Echinacea produced results showing that around 29 percent of the patients reported a decrease in fatigue. This is not the magic bullet for your fatigue problems, but it might just give you relief. While it is generally safe, it is advised that one should not take it when they want to sleep. An allowance of three hours before sleep is usually indicated as it can keep you up.

Possible side effects: Stomach aches, minor difficulty sleeping, possible allergic reactions

- **Green Tea**

Green tea is as well recognized as Chamomile tea and is widely used by many. It also holds benefits for those with Fibromyalgia. Green tea can give a person a boost in energy and can decrease pain and feelings of fatigue. However, it has to be noted that this is not usually advisable for people who are already having trouble sleeping as it often used to keep people awake and alert.

Possible side effects: (if not taken in moderation) Upset stomach, anxiety, increased blood pressure, insomnia. It is also known to counter the effects of anti-clotting medication.

Oils, Ointments and Essences

Some of the common FMS remedies being used are those that are actually applied on to your skin. These are known as topical remedies and many of them are actually derived from plants themselves. Whether it is oils or ointments, the ingredients for these are straight from nature, often making them cheap due to the decrease in processing cost.

Here are some of the commonly used remedies. Many of them are ingredients in sprays and ointments so read the labels:

- **Capsaicin**

    It is an oil derived from chili peppers. It is used as an anesthetic. Applying it on skin reduces the chemicals that fire of the pain signals to your brain. Be careful when using it as it can irritate your eyes.

- **Eucalyptus**

    It is derived from the leaves that cuddly koalas also happen to eat. It is a mild stimulant and when applied to skin, it relieves tensed muscles, allowing them to relax.

- **Cayenne**

    This also comes from hot peppers. It causes your skin to heat up and relaxes you muscles.

- **Peppermint oil**

    This is a common flavoring for food, but it can also be used as a topical painkiller.

- **Methyl salicylate**

    This is a derivative of aspirin. Found in many plant sources, it is both an anesthetic and a painkiller. However, since it is based on aspirin, it can cause the same stomach problems even if it is applied to the skin.

- **Menthol**

  It is much like eucalyptus. While it is known for its aroma, if applied to skin or strained muscles, it gives temporary pain relief.

There are many other similar natural and herbal ingredients that can help with pain. You can ask your doctor about them.

Chapter 3 – Alternative Therapies

With all the pain and muscle tension, many who suffer FMS may be reluctant to have someone touch them and apply pressure to their muscles and skin. However, as far as natural remedies go, hands-on therapies are actually well received by both patients and medical practitioners. There have been many recorded successes with the use of the following therapy methods in alleviating pain and tension. They might even be the first things suggested by your physician aside from medication. Here is a brief overview of the most common types of hands-on therapy that you can try:

- **Heat Therapy**

  This is often cited as the most preferred of the hands-on remedies. It has been used to treat patients with chronic pain even before it was used for patients with FMS. It is based on the idea that heat helps promote blood flow in the area where it is applied. So when heat is applied where there is pain, the increase in blood flow makes it heal faster as well as relaxes tense muscles.

- **Hydrotherapy or Water Therapy**

  No, this is not therapy involving drinking water. Instead, it makes use of exercise and massage while submerged in water. Those with muscle injuries, as well those undergoing physical therapy, often use this kind of therapy. Stretching and aerobic activities in the water help one relax and release tension in the muscles. The water provides slight support, giving the person a partial weightlessness. This can be done in your own pool or even in your hot tub. The temperature of the water can also be adjusted for specific desired effects. Aside from relieving pain, it has also been known to help with insomnia. You can probably relate if you have ever dozed off in a bathtub filled with warm water.

- **Cold Therapy**

  This therapy is very similar to heat therapy, but uses cold instead. The idea is that cold dulls the sensation of pain. It numbs the nerves and prevents them from transmitting the mixed up pain signals. It is also used to stop inflammation by slowing down the flow of blood. This is often used for cases of acute pain and not chronic pain, but it can help some of those who are suffering from FMS. Be careful when using this therapy as some FMS patients have been known to be sensitive to cold. This might just worsen the pain for some.

- **Massage Therapy**

  This is the most mainstream of hands-on therapies, but it is also the one which makes patients cringe a lot. Unlike the others already mentioned, this involves applying pressure to parts of the body. This does not sound good for FMS patients when one of the main symptoms they suffer is sensitivity to pressure. On good days, however, it might be a good idea to try this therapy to help relax your muscles.

This therapy is also good for releasing your mental tension and can help cope with "fibro-fog". It encourages you to let go of your stress and anxiety so it not only helps with your body, but also your mind. This can also be used alongside heat and cold therapy for increased effect. Just be sure that your massage therapist understands your condition and is careful enough to listen when you are in pain.

Chapter 4 – Focusing On Your Body and Mind

Fibromyalgia is more than a condition that affects your body. FMS is all about a miscommunication of your body and your central nervous system. It also involves mental confusion and a lot of stress and anxiety. So it only makes sense that when treating FMS, one must find a balance between body and mind. Here are some methods that FMS patients have tried:

Relaxation Therapy

This is all about calming both your mind and body through use of willpower and intention. This might sound like a lot to ask, but it is actually quite simple. All you have to do is to concentrate on your body part or an area. While you keep your concentration, you intentionally relax this area. You do this moving from one muscle to another, one body part to the next until your whole body is relaxed. You look for a therapist offering relaxation therapy or you can even do it yourself.

Here are instructions you can follow on your own:

1. Find a dim area you can use. Darkness can help you relax like when you go to sleep.

2. Put yourself in a comfortable position preferably lying down.

3. Begin focusing on your body. Start with a body part or a single muscle.

4. Control your breathing and slow it down. As you do, visualize your muscle or body part starting to relax. Think of it tensing up then releasing. Do this until it is relaxed.

5. Continue this by progressing from one muscle to another systematically. Only move on to the next when one muscle is relaxed.

Meditation

Meditation is also a common form of therapy that is utilized by several therapists for pain related conditions. It comes in several forms and if you tried the instructions above, you have just been introduced to a simple form of meditation. The main concept behind this is to utilize your ability to focus in order to divert your attention from your pain, stress and anxiety. Some other forms do not let you ignore them, but instead face them so you can deal with them head on. Using meditation is known to help with pain, sleeping problems as well as fibro-fog. This is not a quick fix or a sure fire way to deal with FMS, but it has been producing positive results. It is a perfect way of synchronizing your body and your mind.

As mentioned, there are several options for you if you want to try meditation. You can approach clinical therapists who offer guided meditation. It is also possible to join meditation classes. It can also be as simple as finding instructions online or picking up a book on practical meditation. Once you get the hang of it, you will be able to practice it on your own in the comfort of your home.

Yoga

Yoga is also a popular option for people who suffer from conditions that involve muscle pain and chronic pain. It is more than likely that you are imagining people contorting their bodies and thinking how painful that might be. Well you have been misled by the stereotypes shown on television. Yoga is not about putting your legs behind your head or doing extreme feats of flexibility. While many advance practitioners do exhibit great control of their bodies to the extent of having very flexible bodies, practical yoga does not focus on this at all. Practical yoga is all about developing control over both body and mind. This is done by learning breathing and stretching techniques blended with meditation. This creates a stronger link between the body and the mind and can help you deal with pain, fatigue and even confusion. Other than that, it is also a good form of exercise to keep you in shape.

Exercise

One other thing for you to try is good old fashioned exercise. If you have visited a doctor about FMS, then this might have been already suggested to you. If not, you can expect it. You may be thinking that with all the pain and fatigue you are feeling, exercise is out of the question. However, doctors, therapists and even FMS patients who exercise all swear by it. Exercise when properly monitored and programmed has been proven to aid persons with muscle injuries and chronic muscles pain. For that reason alone, it is a useful tool for managing FMS. Other than that, exercise is also a key to maintaining proper homeostasis, which makes sure that you get enough sleep when you need it.

Another warning is in order here. Remember that you should not just rush to the gym and start lifting weights. Considering you condition, you have to make sure that you do the right kinds of exercise with the right kind of guidance. For your benefit, here are some important tips when considering exercise:

- Find an exercise program that fits your present condition. Slow and light is a good place to start. You are trying to avoid pain and not cause more.

- Do not set unrealistic goals. Be clear with yourself about what you can do and what you cannot while considering your condition. There is no shame in admitting that you are not able to do some things like you did before. Make this clear with your fitness coach or therapist as well so they do not end up getting you hurt.

- Take note that you should avoid static exercises and instead focus on dynamic ones. This means you should try not to lift weights, but instead try walking, jogging or swimming. This is because lifting weights can cause more pain than relief for FMS patients.

- Always consult a professional. Do not rely on something you have seen online or on TV without making sure it will not hurt you in some way.

- Take your time and be patient. Slow and steady treats Fibromyalgia. You must not get frustrated if you are not up and running immediately. This is a treatment and not a competition. You need to push yourself a bit to get started, but not too much to worsen the pain and cause more grief.

Chapter 5 – Beating the Fibro-Fog

Fibro-fog is probably the most unique symptom that is associated with Fibromyalgia. Research has been done on the symptom and it points towards sleep deprivation and even depression as the cause of the confusion and lack of focus. Other research refutes this saying that a lack of oxygen to the brain caused by the malfunctioning nervous system makes one unfocused and feeling off. In reality, it would be hard to distinguish which part of the symptom would be caused by a sleep deficit or from your faulty brain wiring. Nevertheless, you are not without solutions.

The following are simple tips and tricks to keep you on point despite the Fibro-Fog. The great thing is that they are all practical and all natural.

- **Stay away from tough tasks when you are in pain (or tired).**

  It is and obvious thing to say but many still forget this. When you are feeling out of focus and confused, you tend to be less capable of dealing with the pain. Well this works both ways as well. When you are in pain and fatigued, you will be less likely to think clearly after. Add to this the effects of Fibro-Fog and it becomes a vicious cycle of pain and confusion. When you are tired and in pain, do not push yourself too hard. Know your limitations, but don't drop all your responsibilities. Strike a proper balance.

- **Getting help from others.**

If you are experiencing the "fog" on a regular basis, whether it is at home or at work, then you might consider finding a buddy to help you. At home, you can ask your spouse or even children to help you out when the fog comes in. At work, you can ask a buddy of yours to remind you of important tasks or simply to get back your focus. Ask them to give you tiny signals like a tap on the shoulder or maybe a word when you seem to be drifting off. Just make sure to explain to them the nature of your condition.

- **Making full use of lists.**

Many successful people swear by the amazing habit of making lists and plans. It keeps them focused and on point when they have many things to do and all of them are important. If you have FMS, you can see how useful this can be. It can remind you of what you have to do and it might even improve your performance at work or at home and make you more efficient than a person without FMS.

Just remember, however, that you should not overload your lists. Remember the first item above. Do not overwork yourself as this will likely worsen your fogginess.

- **Sleeping right.**

Sleeping is very important if you want to maintain your focus. Aside from its restorative function, it also helps you keep your concentration and calm. It is not just about resting your aches and calming your mind. While you sleep, your body releases hormones and neurochemicals that help keep you functional both in body and mind. If you skip this important part by losing sleep, you are essentially losing some bodily functions. This may aggravate the Fibro-fog or even be its main cause. At any rate, if you have FMS and you have sleeping problems, you should ask your doctor for treatment for this immediately. You will notice a great change in your disposition once you get enough sleep.

- **Making full use of a calendar.**

This is more or less the same as making lists, but in a larger scale. This is useful for keeping appointments and not worrying about remembering them while you deal with immediate tasks. You can also combine lists and calendars in a daily planner, but some people find this too rigid. Make sure that you place your planned appointments on a calendar that is hard to miss so that even if you are having a bad day, you will never fail to attend a meeting or a doctor's appointment perhaps.

- **Being careful with your diet.**

As your doctor will probably tell you, food has a very potent effect on your mind. It can either boost you or slow you down. Food is just a bunch of substances and chemicals after all. Ask your doctor for any dietary suggestions if you can be bothered. Know which foods can do what. For example, milk and turkey can actually help you with your sleeping problems. Also, caffeine and sugar can worsen fibro-fog by making you anxious and agitated.

- **Getting organized.**

  If you have ever watched great multi-taskers at work, you will notice that they always seem distracted, but they still get a lot of work done. Their secret to this efficiency under pressure is organization. No matter how much they have to do at one time, no matter how distracted they are, if they know where their things are, they will get the work done easier. You can achieve the same effect if you take a leaf from their page and start creating an organized system for the things that you need. Do not clutter your work desk or even your home. Keep important things handy and get rid of things that will only add to the confusion.

- **Monitoring yourself when things get foggy.**

  Your best ally when Fibro-fog hits is yourself. Aside from others helping you, you can also train yourself to catch yourself when you start slipping. One of the most common ways to do this is to give yourself a sort of wake-up call every hour or so. You can achieve this by setting gentler alarms on your phone. Some even resort to watches that beep every hour or so. This is great for snapping yourself out of the fog when no one is there with you.

Conclusion

Thank you again for downloading this book!

I hope this book has given you the important information you need about Fibromyalgia. With the information on natural and alternative remedies contained here, you should be well equipped to deal with Fibromyalgia the natural way.

Now that you are on your way to recovery, the next step for you is to explore new remedies being developed as well as the growing amount of research on the condition.

Thank you and good luck!